Nosebleeds During Pregnancy

Causes and Remedies

Dr, Tiffany J. Bozeman

CONTENTS

- <u>Emotional Support for Pregnant Women Suffering from Nosebleeds</u>
- <u>Strategies for Handling Stress and Anxiety Caused by Nosebleeds</u>
- <u>Coping Techniques for Pregnancy-Related Nosebleeds</u>

CHAPTER ONE

Introduction

Many women worry about nosebleeds since they happen often during pregnancy. It's critical to comprehend the causes, dangers, and treatment options for nosebleeds throughout pregnancy. In this chapter, we'll examine the nose's structure, the definition of a nosebleed, the reasons why pregnant women have them, and the dangers of nosebleeds.

The Anatomy Of The Nose

The nose is a fundamental organ that is in charge of the sense of smell and is also essential for breathing. The external nose, nasal septum, nasal cavity, and sinuses are just a few of the components that make up the nose. What we can see of the exterior of the nose is formed of bone and cartilage. The wall between the two nostrils is called the nasal septum, and it is formed of bone and cartilage. The mucosa, a thin layer of tissue, lines the nasal cavity, a space within the nose. The face's bones include cavities called sinuses that are filled with air.

What Exactly Is A Nosebleed?

Blood that has leaked from the blood vessels in the nose's lining is known as a nosebleed. Anterior and posterior nosebleeds are two different varieties. Blood vessels at the front of the nose burst, causing more frequent anterior nosebleeds. Less often occurring posterior nosebleeds result from a rupture of the blood vessels at the back of the nose.

What Causes Nosebleeds in Pregnant Women

For a variety of reasons, pregnant women are more likely to get nosebleeds. The nasal mucosa's blood vessels may become more fragile and more prone to rupture due to hormonal changes that take place during pregnancy. The strain on the blood vessels in the nose caused by the increased blood volume during pregnancy might potentially increase the risk of nosebleeds. Moreover, the increased blood flow to the nose's mucous membranes might enlarge them and make them more vulnerable to bleeding.

Pregnancy-Related Nosebleed Risk Factors

Nosebleeds during pregnancy are more likely when several risk factors are present. These risk elements consist of:

1. Dry air: Dry air may aggravate and dry up the nasal mucosa, increasing the likelihood of nosebleeds.

2. High altitude: High altitude may make the blood vessels in the nose enlarge, which raises the possibility of nosebleeds.

3. Nasal congestion: Nasal congestion might increase the susceptibility of the blood vessels in the nose to rupturing.

4. Trauma: When the nose is injured, the blood vessels may burst, resulting in a nosebleed.

5. Allergies: Allergies may irritate the nasal mucosa and increase the likelihood of nosebleeds.

To properly treat nosebleeds during pregnancy, you must first understand why they happen. Due to hormonal changes, increased blood volume, and increased blood flow to the nasal mucosa, pregnant women are more likely to have nosebleeds. Nasal congestion, trauma, allergies, dry air, and high altitude, and these risk factors may all increase the probability of nosebleeds during pregnancy. Women may take proactive steps to avoid and control nosebleeds during pregnancy by being aware of the causes and risk factors connected with them.

Nosebleed Complications During Pregnancy

While nosebleeds are normal during pregnancy, they may sometimes be concerning. Although nosebleeds are often not harmful, if they are not managed, they might cause difficulties. The dangers of nosebleeds during pregnancy, when to seek medical help, and how they might influence your pregnancy are all covered in this chapter.

How and when to seek medical help

The majority of nosebleeds that occur during pregnancy are mild and manageable at home. But, in certain circumstances, getting medical help is necessary. Consider getting medical help if:

1. You get a severe nosebleed that lasts for more than 20 minutes.

2. You have blood clots or significant bleeding.

3. You feel faint, lightheaded, or woozy.

4. Breathing is tough for you.

5. You get palpitations or discomfort in your chest.

6. You have a terrible headache or clouded vision.

Common Nosebleed Problems During Pregnancy

Although most nosebleeds that occur during pregnancy are innocuous, if they are not addressed, they might cause difficulties. Common nosebleed issues during pregnancy include the following:

1. Anemia, a disorder marked by a low quantity of red blood cells in the body, may result from nosebleeds. Shortness of breath, weakness, and exhaustion are all symptoms of anemia.

2. Preterm labor: Nosebleeds may result in the release of the hormone oxytocin, which can start labor contractions.

3. Fetal discomfort may result from a drop in the fetus's oxygen supply, which can be brought on by severe nosebleeds.

4. Nosebleeds might raise your chance of getting illnesses like sinus infections or pneumonia.

The Effects of Nosebleeds on Pregnancy

Pregnancy nosebleeds may be concerning, particularly if they result in difficulties. Your pregnancy may be impacted by nosebleeds in several ways, including:

1. Recurrent nosebleeds may be worrisome and anxious, which can have an impact on your mental health while pregnant.

2. Nosebleeds may be painful and uncomfortable, which might lower your quality of life during pregnancy.

3. Regular nosebleeds might cause you to engage in less physical activity, which can negatively impact your pregnancy's general health.

4. Complications are more likely as a result of nosebleeds during pregnancy, including anemia, premature labor, and decreased oxygen to the baby.

If ignored, nosebleeds during pregnancy might result in difficulties. If you get severe nosebleeds or any other symptoms like dizziness, chest discomfort, or trouble breathing, you must visit a doctor right away. Anemia, premature labor, decreased fetal oxygenation, and infections are common side effects of nosebleeds during pregnancy. Your pregnancy may also be impacted by nosebleeds since they may be stressful, uncomfortable, and cause you to be less active. You may take proactive steps to avoid and successfully manage nosebleeds during pregnancy by being aware of the possible side effects.

CHAPTER TWO

Controlling Nasal Bleeds During Pregnancy

While nosebleeds during pregnancy might be concerning, they are often treatable at home. The self-care techniques and home remedies you may employ to treat nosebleeds while pregnant are covered in this chapter. We will also talk about over-the-counter drugs and nasal saline sprays that may help treat nosebleed symptoms.

Self-Care Techniques for Pregnancy-Related Nosebleeds

There are various self-care techniques you may do to stop bleeding if you get a nosebleed while pregnant, including:

1. Pinch your nose: Hold the pinch for 10 to 15 minutes, right below the bony section.

2. Lean slightly forward and squeeze your nose to stop the blood from running down your throat.

3. Use ice: To assist constrict the blood vessels and halt the bleeding, apply an ice

pack or a cold compress on the bridge of your nose.

4. The healing process might be slowed down and the bleeding can intensify if you blow your nose.

5. Maintaining enough hydration might help prevent nosebleeds by keeping your nasal passages wet.

Natural Treatments for Nosebleeds

You may employ a variety of home remedies to treat nosebleeds while pregnant, including:

1. Saline solution: Rinsing your nasal passages with saline solution helps keep them moist and lessen the likelihood of nosebleeds.

2. Use a humidifier to maintain moisture in the air in your house and stop your nasal passages from drying out.

3. Vitamin C: Oranges and kiwis are two foods high in vitamin C that may help strengthen your blood vessels and lower your risk of nosebleeds.

4. Essential oils: Eucalyptus and lavender are two essential oils that might help calm

your nasal passages and lessen the likelihood of nosebleeds.

Medicines available over the counter

You may treat the symptoms of nosebleeds with several over-the-counter drugs, including:

1.   Nasal decongestants: Nasal decongestants may assist lessen nasal congestion and stop nosebleeds. Examples include phenylephrine and oxymetazoline.

2. Antihistamines: Antihistamines may lessen nasal irritation and stop

nosebleeds. Examples include loratadine and cetirizine.

3. Supplemental vitamin K: Vitamin K may help strengthen your blood vessels and lower your risk of bleeding from the nose.

Saline Nasal Sprays:

Nasal saline sprays are a secure and efficient technique to treat nosebleed symptoms when pregnant. They function by hydrating your nasal cavities and lowering the possibility of nosebleeds. The following are a few advantages of utilizing nasal saline sprays:

1. Nasal saline sprays are safe for pregnant women and may be used at any time throughout pregnancy.

2. Nasal saline sprays don't have any negative effects, and it's unlikely that they will interfere with other drugs.

3. Simple administration: Nasal saline sprays are simple to use and may be used at home.

Nasal saline sprays, over-the-counter drugs, home treatments, and self-care techniques may all be used to treat nosebleeds while pregnant. Leaning forward, squeezing your nose, and using ice, among other self-care techniques, may halt the bleeding. Saline solutions, humidifiers, vitamin C, and essential oils are examples of natural therapies that may help lower the incidence of nosebleeds. The symptoms of nosebleeds may be controlled with over-the-counter drugs such as nasal decongestants, antihistamines, and vitamin K supplements. Inhaled saline

Avoiding Nosebleeds When Pregnant

For expectant women, nosebleeds during pregnancy may be painful and worrying. It is usually preferable to avoid them in the first place, even if they may be treated with the right remedies. We will go over some advice for avoiding nosebleeds during pregnancy in this chapter. We will also discuss several healthy practices expecting mothers may take to lower their chance of nosebleeds, as well as some typical triggers to stay away from.

Guidelines for Preventing Nosebleeds During Pregnancy

1. Keep your nasal passages wet: Maintaining a moist nasal channel is one of the best strategies to avoid nosebleeds

during pregnancy. A humidifier, a warm shower, or a saline nose spray may all help with this.

2. Drink lots of water to stay hydrated: This will keep your nasal passages wet and stop them from drying out. Aim for 8 to 10 glasses of water every day, minimum.

3. Avoid blowing your nose too forcefully since it might irritate your nasal passages and increase your chance of getting a nosebleed. Instead, try softly blowing your nose or using a nasal aspirator.

4. Avoid picking your nose, using abrasive tissues, or cotton swabs to clean it. Be careful while doing so. They may irritate some and result in nosebleeds.

5. Consider employing a nasal filter if you are allergic to or sensitive to pollutants to keep them out of your nasal passages.

Healthy Practices for Expectant Women

Pregnancy-related healthy behaviors may help lower the risk of nosebleeds. Pregnant women may adopt the following healthy behaviors:

1. Maintain a healthy diet: Eating a balanced, nutrient-rich diet will assist your blood vessels to get stronger and lower your risk of nosebleeds. Have a diet rich in whole grains, lean proteins, fruits, and vegetables.

2. Frequent exercise helps strengthen your blood vessels and increase circulation, lowering your risk of nosebleeds.

3. Get adequate sleep: Sleep is essential for general health and may help lower stress, which can cause nosebleeds.

4. Control your stress: Stress might make nosebleeds during pregnancy more likely. Think about engaging in relaxation methods like yoga, meditation, or deep breathing.

Avoid Common Triggers:

Pregnant women should avoid several frequent triggers to lower their risk of nosebleeds. A few of them are:

1. Dry air: Dry air may cause nosebleeds by irritating the nasal passages. To maintain moisture in your home's air, use a humidifier.

2. Allergens: Allergens may irritate the nasal passages and raise the risk of nosebleeds. Examples of these allergens include pollen, dust, and pet dander. As much as you can, keep away from these allergens' exposure.

3. Irritants: Being around irritants like smoke, chemicals, and strong scents might make it more likely that you will get nosebleeds. Try to limit your exposure to these irritants.

4. Medication: Aspirin and blood thinners, for example, may raise the risk of nosebleeds. Before beginning any new

drug while pregnant, see your healthcare practitioner.

By forming healthy habits, avoiding frequent triggers, and maintaining moist nasal passages, nosebleeds during pregnancy may be avoided. Keep yourself hydrated, refrain from blowing your nose too forcefully, and use a nasal filter as a prevention strategy for nosebleeds. Pregnant women should practice healthy behaviors including eating a balanced diet, working out often, getting adequate sleep, and controlling their stress. Avoiding dry air, allergies, irritants, and certain drugs are some common causes. You may lessen your risk of nosebleeds and have a safe pregnancy by implementing these suggestions and good lifestyle choices.

CHAPTER THREE

Options For Treating Nosebleeds During Pregnant

For expectant women, nosebleeds during pregnancy may be painful and worrying. Despite your best efforts, nosebleeds may still happen even though there are several strategies to avoid them. We will look at the many alternatives for treating nosebleeds during pregnancy in this chapter. We'll go over medication remedies for controlling nosebleeds as well as possible surgical solutions for more serious situations.

Medicinal Solutions for Pregnancy-Related Nosebleeds

1. Applying direct pressure to the bleeding nostril is one of the most efficient techniques to stop a nosebleed. Pinch your nostrils together with your fingers for 10 to 15 minutes to do this.

2. Nasal sprays: Over-the-counter nasal sprays may assist decrease nasal passageway irritation and stop nosebleeds. These sprays include saline solution, which may aid in maintaining the moisture of the nasal passages.

3. Silver nitrate is a substance that may be put into the region that is bleeding to assist in stopping the bleeding. The usual setting for this therapy is a medical office or clinic.

4. Cauterization: With a hot device, bleeding blood vessels are burnt or cauterized during this process. This is a more intrusive therapeutic option that is often performed under local anesthetic. Surgical Techniques for Serious Conditions

To control nosebleeds during pregnancy, surgical treatments may be required in extreme circumstances. Some of these techniques consist of:

1. Endoscopic surgery: Endoscopic surgery includes seeing into the nasal passages with a camera mounted on a thin, flexible tube. This enables the surgeon to find and address the bleeding's origin.

2. Packing: In certain circumstances, it may be required to halt the bleeding by packing the nasal passages with gauze or other materials. Usually performed under local anesthetic, this might need hospitalization.

3. Embolization is a minimally invasive technique that involves injecting tiny particles into the blood vessels that are responsible for the nosebleed. This reduces bleeding by obstructing blood flow to the location.

Many medicinal and surgical methods may be used to address nosebleeds during pregnancy. Direct pressure, nasal sprays, silver nitrate, and cauterization are examples of medical therapies. Surgery techniques such as packing, embolization, and endoscopic surgery may be required in extreme situations. It's crucial to contact a doctor if you have frequent or severe nosebleeds while pregnant to identify the underlying reason and the most appropriate course of action. You may control your nosebleeds and have a safe pregnancy by collaborating with your healthcare professional.

How To Manage Nosebleeds When Pregnant

Expectant moms may experience discomfort if they have frequent or severe nosebleeds during pregnancy. Dealing with the emotional effects that nosebleeds may have on your mental health and wellness is an important part of coping with nosebleeds in addition to treating the physical symptoms. We will look at several coping mechanisms in this chapter to help you deal with nosebleeds while pregnant.

Emotional Support for Pregnant Women Suffering from Nosebleeds

Emotional support is one of the most crucial components of managing nosebleeds during pregnancy. This may come from your spouse, family, friends, or medical professionals, among other people. It is important to express your feelings to others and to request assistance when necessary.

Seeking the assistance of a mental health expert may be beneficial if you are going through severe emotional anguish as a result of nosebleeds during pregnancy. These professionals may be therapists, counselors, or psychologists who can provide you with the instruments and coping mechanisms you need to deal with your emotions.

Strategies for Handling Stress and Anxiety Caused by Nosebleeds

Expectant moms may experience tension and anxiety due to nosebleeds, particularly if they are severe or frequent.

You may use several techniques to deal with stress and worry caused by nosebleeds, including:

1. Focusing your attention on the present moment without passing judgment is a component of mindfulness meditation. You may enhance your general mental health and lessen the tension and worry that comes with nosebleeds by doing this.

2. Exercise: Frequent exercise will help you feel less stressed and anxious and will also benefit your physical health in general. Discuss safe exercise alternatives with your healthcare physician while you are pregnant.

3. Deep breathing, gradual muscle relaxation, and visualization are just a few relaxation methods that might help you feel less stressed and anxious.

Coping Techniques for Pregnancy-Related Nosebleeds

You may utilize a variety of coping mechanisms, such as the ones listed below, in addition to emotional support and stress reduction measures, to cope with nosebleeds during pregnancy, including:

1. Maintain a record: Keep track of when your nosebleeds happen, how long they persist, and any potential causes. This might assist you in seeing trends and modifying your everyday habits to lessen the frequency of nosebleeds.

2. Maintaining enough hydration can assist to keep your nasal passages wet and lower the chance of nosebleeds.

3. Employ a humidifier: Keeping the air moist in your house using a humidifier may help lower the risk of nosebleeds.

4. Prevent triggers: Steer clear of substances like alcohol, dry air, and irritants that might cause nosebleeds.

Conclusion

Dealing with the emotional effects that nosebleeds might have on your mental health and wellness is just as important as treating the physical symptoms of nosebleeds during pregnancy. You can control nosebleeds and have a safe pregnancy with the use of emotional support, stress-reduction methods, and coping mechanisms. You may lessen the frequency and intensity of nosebleeds while using these coping mechanisms in conjunction with your healthcare practitioner, maintaining your general health and welfare during pregnancy.